# Mighty Mind Mantra's For Men

How mantra's, mindfulness and writing therapy, can help you deal with how you feel.

By
Bella Hope Smith

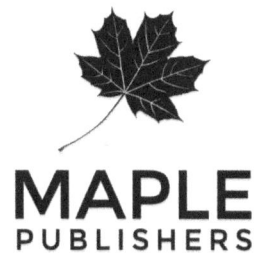

MAPLE
PUBLISHERS

Mighty Mind Mantra's For Men

Author: Bella Hope Smith

Copyright © Bella Hope Smith

The right of Bella Hope Smith to be identified as author of this work has been asserted by the author in accordance with section 77 and 78 of the Copyright, Designs and Patents Act 1988.

First Published in 2025

ISBN 978-1-83538-566-1 (Paperback)

Book Cover, Illustrations, and Book Layout by:
    White Magic Studios
    www.whitemagicstudios.co.uk

Published by:
    Maple Publishers
    Fairbourne Drive, Atterbury,
    Milton Keynes,
    MK10 9RG, UK
    www.maplepublishers.com

A CIP catalogue record for this title is available from the British Library.

All rights reserved. No part of this book may be reproduced or translated by any form or by any means, electronic or mechanical, including photocopying, recording or by any information storage and retrieval system without written permission from the author.

# Introduction

Hello, thank you for buying my book. Mental health is such an important topic. I wanted to write this book, to help you look at different ways of expressing your feelings. Talking about how we feel can be tough sometimes, that is why writing can be another healing tool you can use. In this book I will show you how to write your own healing mantra's, create powerful poems and show you how mindful exercises can help to calm your thoughts too. If you would like to contact me, please email: spirituallypoetical@gmail.com

# Big Benefits of Writing

Firstly, I would like to share some great benefits of writing.

- Reduces stress so you worry less.
- Provides an avenue to express your view.
- Helps with releasing unwanted emotions, so you can set healing in motion.
- Allows room for positive feelings, that provide so much healing.

Writing helps with releasing and opening up hurt and trauma. If you imagine trauma as a rock, it's really tough and hard to break. Now imagine writing therapy as a pick-axe, it slowly chips away at the rock of trauma, allowing deep-rooted pain that you have held onto for years to be worked through and released. Writing therapy isn't a quick fix, but over time it can make a real difference to how you're feeling and how you view every aspect of your life.

Below are some other ways, how writing as a hobby or career can help brighten and lighten your day.

- Blogging
- Author
- Comedy writer
- Song writing
- Poet
- Greeting card verse writer

The list is endless. Whichever type of writing your drawn to, sharing your journey with others will not only help them, but will help you too.

# Writing How You Feel To Heal

The first exercise we are going to do, is just writing how you feel. You can just write words, short sentences or as much as you want. Don't pressure yourself that you have to write loads and loads, because even writing down a few words each day, is helping you to express and be in touch with your thoughts and feelings. Create a routine of writing, so that you have an outlet to express how you feel and what you need to release. Begin writing on the next few pages, how you feel, what you think about, or any thoughts or words that need to be expressed or released.

_____
_____
_____
_____
_____
_____
_____
_____
_____
_____
_____
_____
_____

Bella Hope Smith

Mighty Mind Mantra's For Men

Bella Hope Smith

Bella Hope Smith

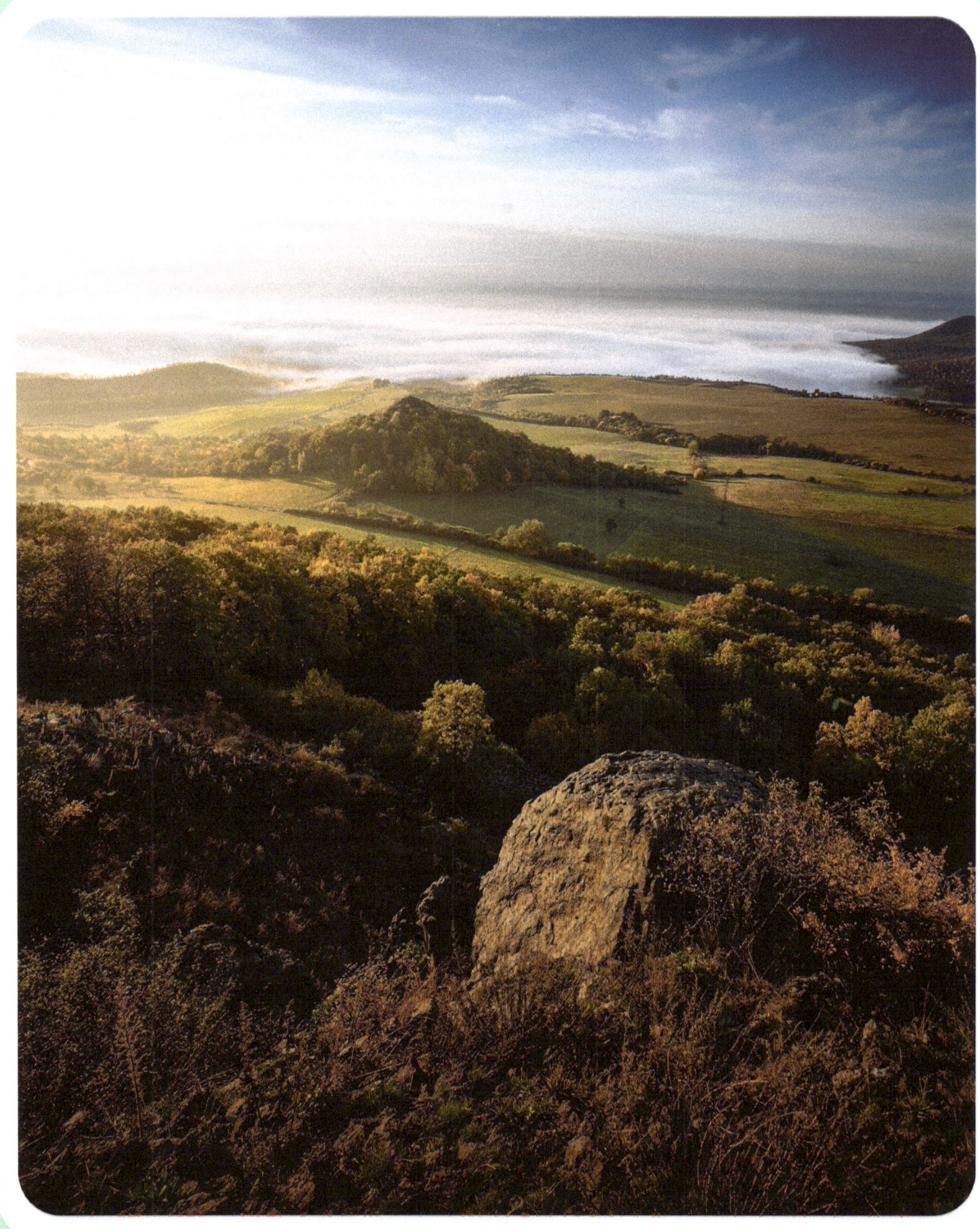

# Explore Feelings Through Drawing

Another tool to help you express how you feel, is through doodling or drawing. Pictures can tell you so much, and is a way to release without saying a word. Drawing can lead to so many things, below is a list of creative paths you could look into to express your feelings through drawing.

- Tattoo artist
- Video game designer
- Greeting card designer
- Architect
- Graphic designer
- Freelance artist
- Product designer
- Watch designer

There are so many creative hobbies and careers you could look into with drawing. On the next few pages, I would like you to express how you feel through doodling or drawing. It doesn't have to be a masterpiece; you can start off with shapes and patterns to get the creativity flowing. You can combine drawing with words too if you like. Try and make doodling or drawing a regular routine too, this will help keep your creative side active and allow you to explore your thoughts and feelings through the way you draw.

Bella Hope Smith

Bella Hope Smith

Bella Hope Smith

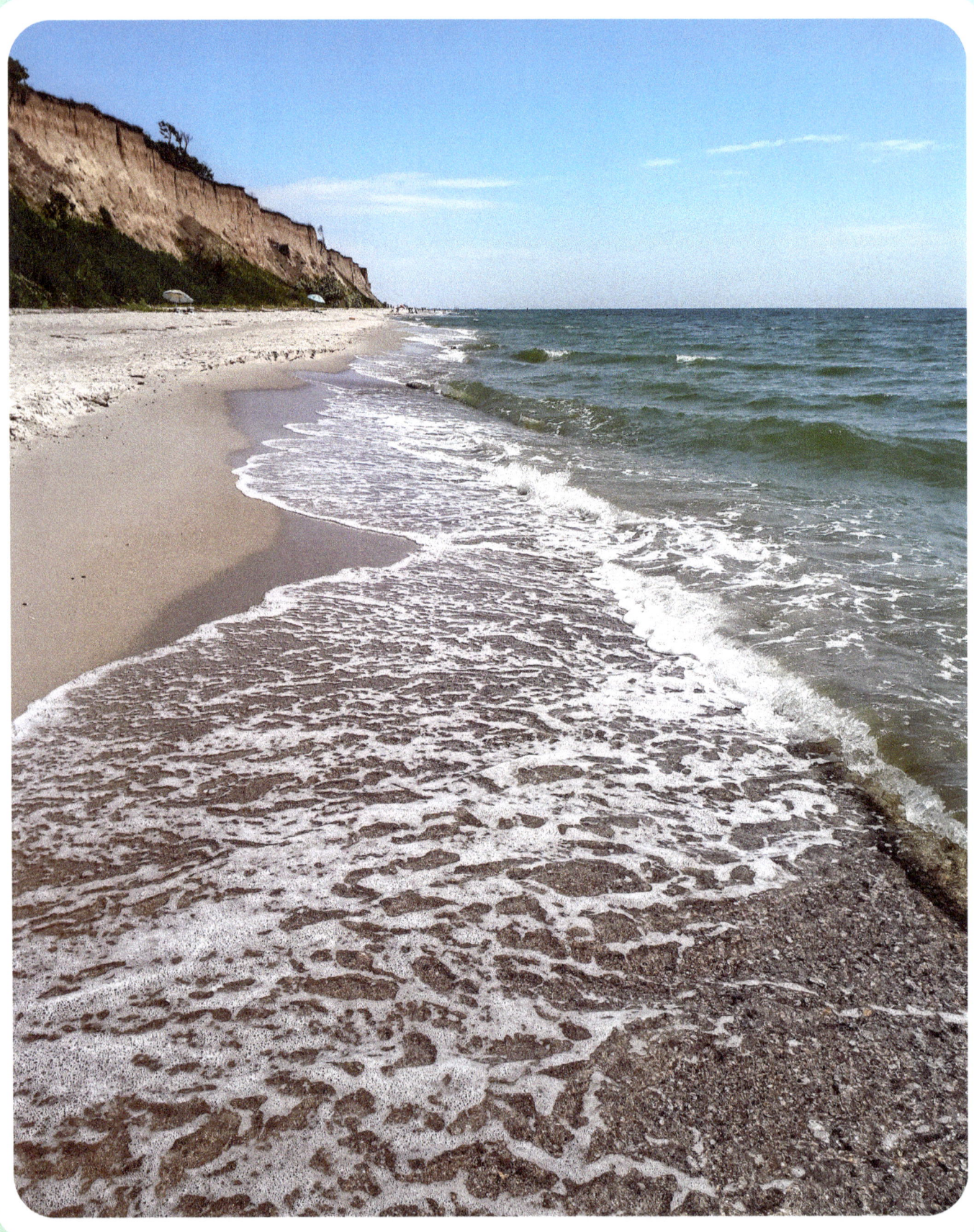

# The Power Of Poetry

Poetry can be very healing, it's a way to put into poetic form what you want to write about in a beautifully healing way. Writing poetry has so many benefits including, helping with expressing emotions, improving creativity, helping improve language skills, creating a calm and therapeutic way of releasing everything, improving self-awareness, boosting mood and so much more.

On the next pages, are a couple of my poems that I have written about mental health. They might resonate and relate to you. Both of my poems are rhymed, but poems don't have to rhyme, it's a way of letting your feelings flow onto paper.

"When everything is hard and you feel like your life is broken,

You pent up your thoughts and feelings, causing them to never be spoken,

Negative emotions keep building and building, getting near to overflowing,

Feeling like this day to day, is really hard to keep going,

It feels like you're in a constant fight,

Where you see no end in sight,

Letting out the baggage that you have had for so long, helps in so many ways,

You will feel better, having much brighter and happier days,

There are lots of ways you can express how you feel; you can talk, sing or write,

Always know you are wanted and worthy. Everything will turn out alright."


"Having a mind full of negative thoughts, is like a dull day that just keeps raining,

Feeling stuck, rageful and depressed makes you feel down and is really draining,

It can make you feel trapped in a cycle that you cannot break,

Filling your mind with such anger, bitterness and hate,

You may want to hide or retreat from life, by putting up a barrier or wall,

Causing you to feel unseen, unheard and like you don't matter at all,

Always know there is someone or something that can help you,

We can help each other; we can make it through."

# Writing Your Own Powerful Poems

I will now show you a technique that you can use to help write your own poems. Remember you don't have to write your poems all in one go. Taking your time and not rushing them, will let you feel more relaxed, allowing the words to flow freely. Below is a technique you can use if you like to help you start off writing poetry.

The first step is choosing a word about a subject that you want to write your poem about.

My example is I am going to choose to create a poem about **Writing**.

Next write the word you have chosen vertically down the page, just like my example below.

W
R
I
T
I
N
G

Now choose some words that describe how you feel about the subject you want to write about, and write them next to each letter of your chosen word, like my example below.

Willpower

Releasing

Inspiration

Transform

Imagination

Nurturing

Grow

The last part is using all the words you have written to describe your subject in your poem. Below is my example I have written.

"With my **willpower** and determination,

I can begin **releasing** any pain that is causing me hurt and aggravation,

I look for creative ways and **inspiration** in all that I do,

So, I can **transform** into the person who I truly want to,

Through writing, my **imagination** runs wild,

Which helps with **nurturing** my soul and inner child,

My mind can now begin to heal and **grow**,

By letting my thoughts and feelings flow".

On the next few pages, try and write your own power poems about anything you like. You can use the technique I just showed you, or you can just let your feelings pour out onto the paper. The technique I showed you, is a way where you have to use words, to describe how you're feeling about your chosen subject you want to write about. Poetry is a really healing way, to express anything you need to say.

Bella Hope Smith

Mighty Mind Mantra's For Men

Bella Hope Smith

# Mighty Mind Mantra's For Men

Mighty Mind Mantra's For Men

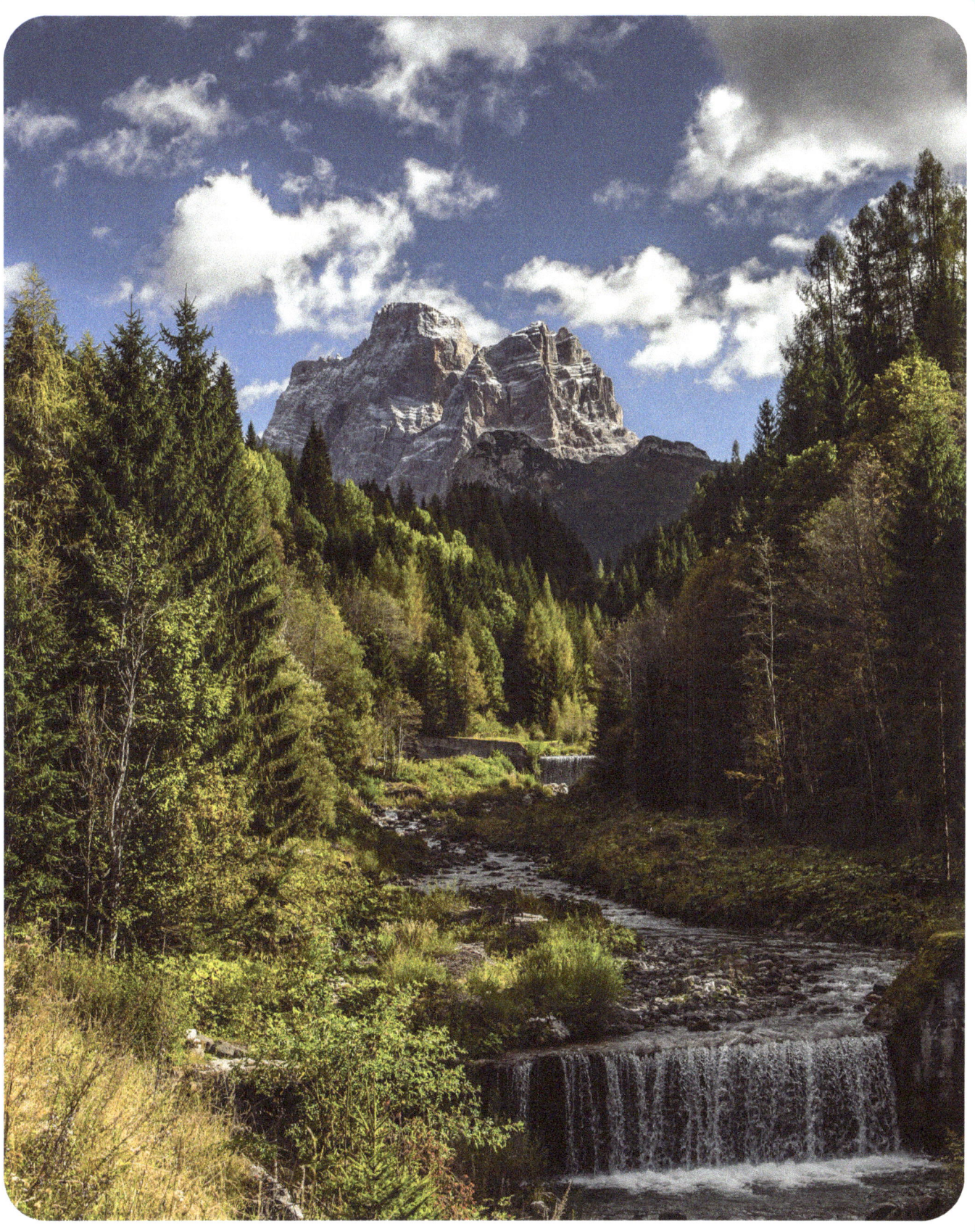

# Picture Poetry

Writing a poem about a picture, is good to get your mind to focus on details of imagery. Look at the picture below or one of the photo's in the book and pick out features that your drawn to. Write in the box on the next page your thoughts and feelings about the picture.

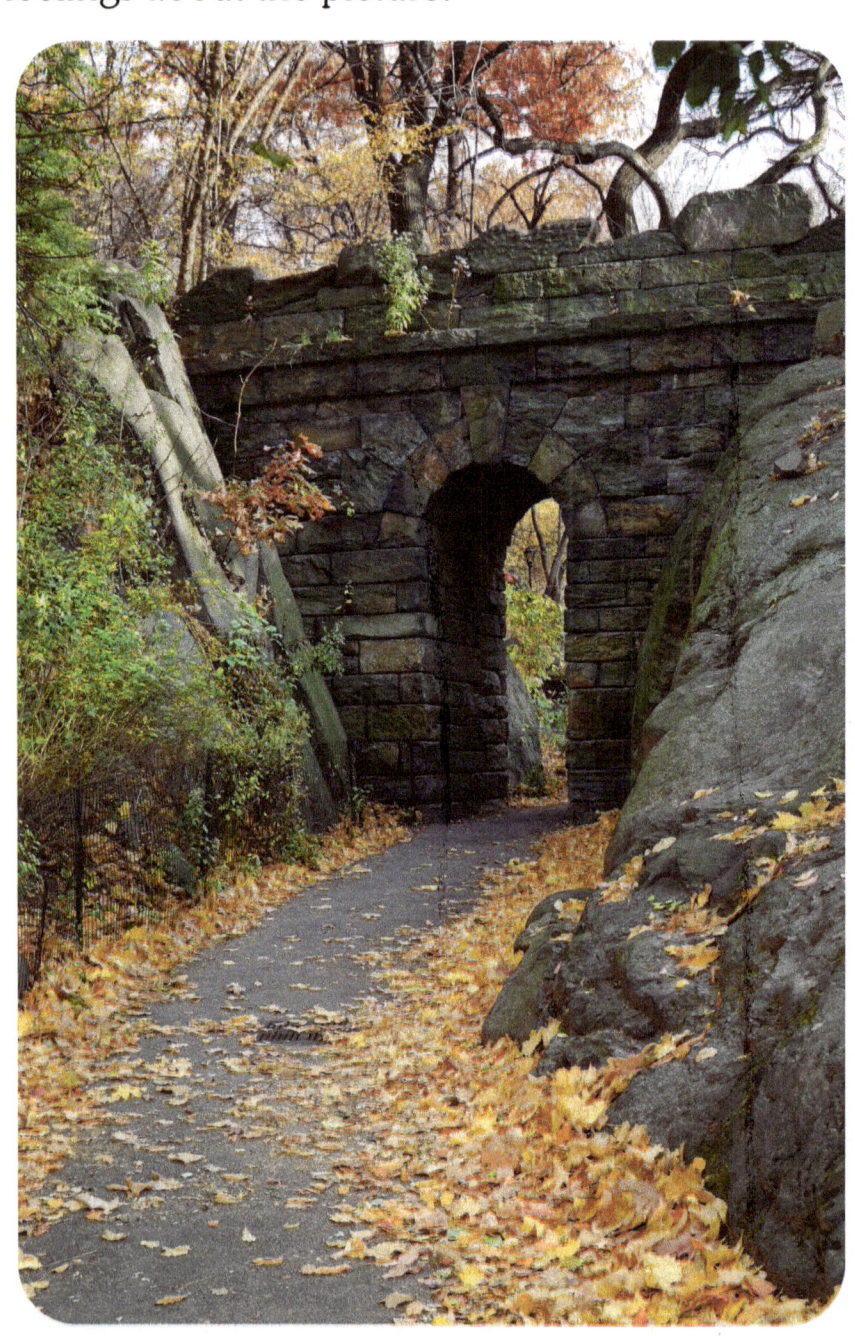

Box to write words and feelings in

Bella Hope Smith

Mighty Mind Mantra's For Men

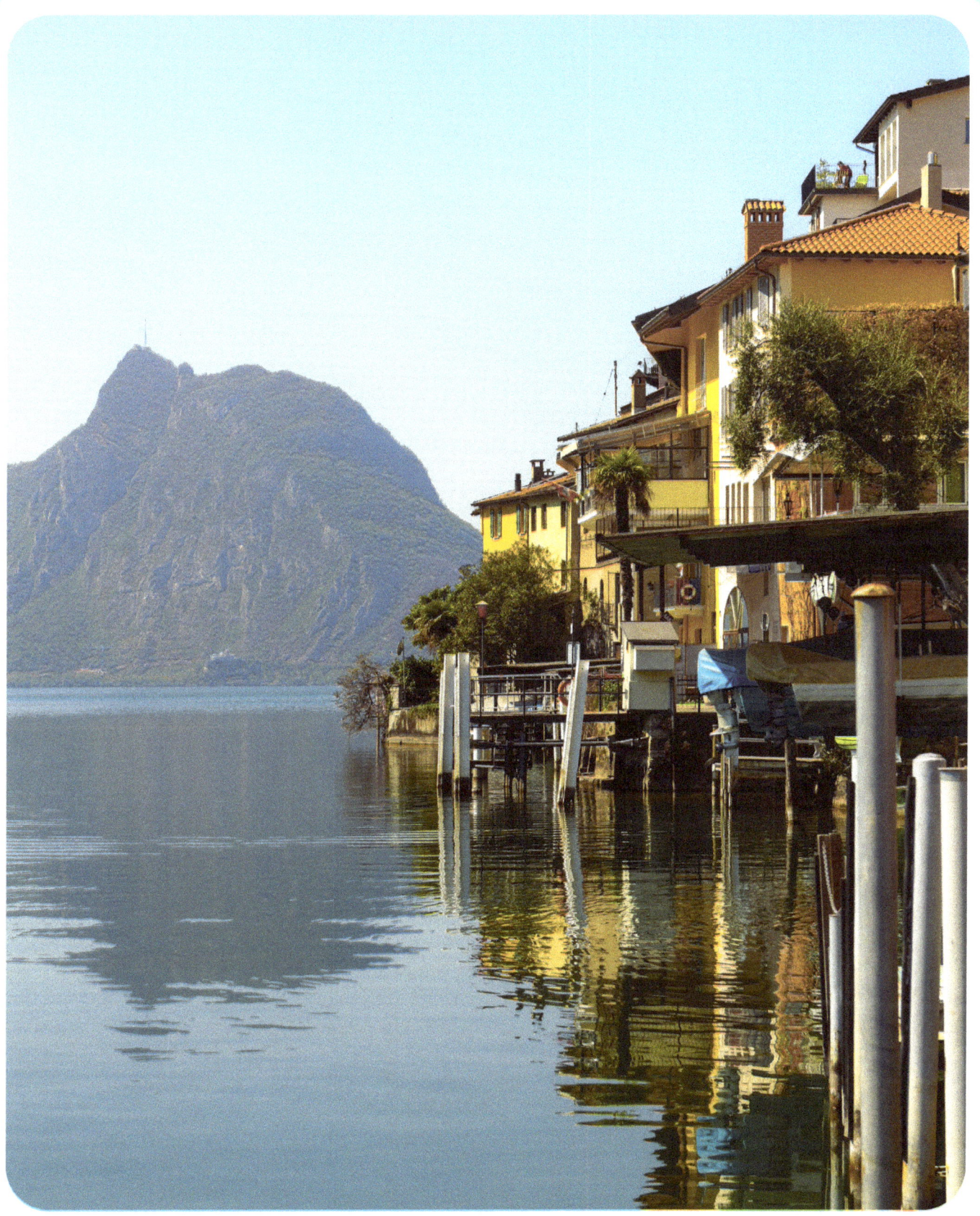

Box to write words and feelings in

Bella Hope Smith

Mighty Mind Mantra's For Men

The next few pages are blank for you to add in your own pictures to write about. You could put a picture of a pet or place in there. You could even go outdoors in your garden, or out for a walk, and take a photo that your drawn to, like a flower garden, scenery, wildlife etc. What would be really powerful, is if you drew your own picture and you write a poem about it. Again, write some describing words and how you feel about the picture in the box below and begin to let your creativity flow.

If you were to add your own picture in the blank frame, it is best to use double sided tape to stick the picture onto the page.

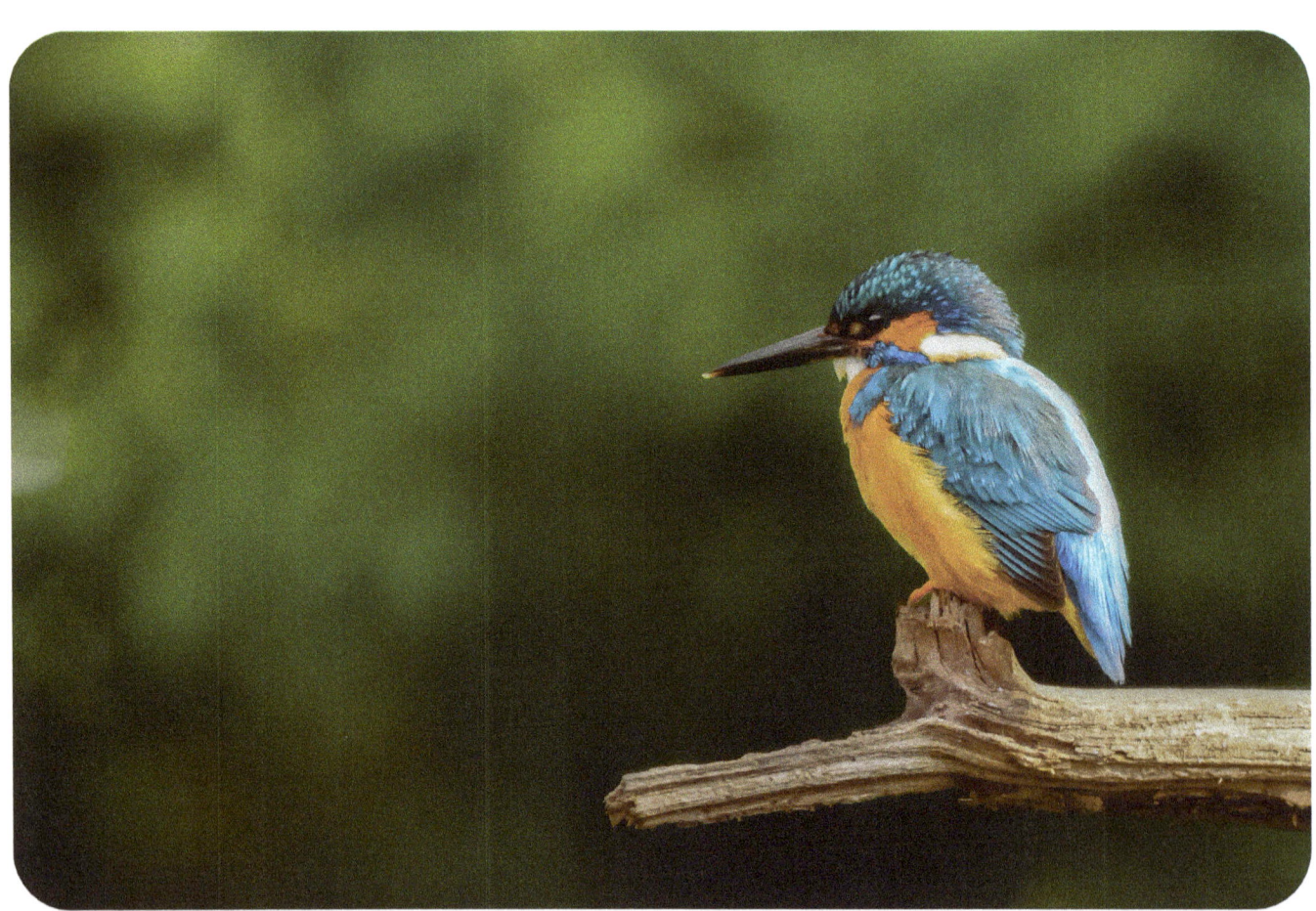

Box to write words and feelings in.

# Mighty Mind Mantra's For Men

Bella Hope Smith

Box to write words and feelings in.

Bella Hope Smith

Mighty Mind Mantra's For Men

Box to write words and feelings in.

Bella Hope Smith

# Mighty Mind Mantra's For Men

# The Magic Of Meditation

Practicing meditation can be really helpful in calming your thoughts, and allowing yourself to take conscious breaths to relax your mind and body.

If you just take some breaths in and out for a few moments, to let your body's system settle down. We are going to do a few exercises that involve keeping your eyes open whilst meditating.

Choose an object to focus on, you can do this inside your house or outdoors.

If your indoors, you could focus on a candle, painting or ornament.

If your outdoors, you could focus on a flower, or nice scenery.

When you have chosen a subject to focus on, take some more deep breaths and start looking at the object, just observing it, whilst taking conscious breaths.

Negative thoughts might pop into your mind, if they do take some more deep breaths and start describing the object you're looking at. This will help distract your mind taking out of negativity and putting your focus on what you're looking at.

If you're looking at a flower, describe the leaves, the petals, the colours etc.

Doing this exercise regularly, will help you when negative thoughts pop in, to take your mind away from spiralling out of control, to bring your awareness back to something more positive.

After doing this exercise I would like you to just take some more deep breaths. Now here comes a bit of colour therapy mixed together with meditation.

With any negative or painful thoughts or feelings that we have, we can alter our energetic systems like the chakra's which are energy points on the body, that can become weak or stuck when negativity floods in. Our aura's are the same, they are energy field's that surround us, and they can become affected from negativity from our thoughts, feelings, emotions and from the outer world too.

Here is an exercise I would like you to try, I have used 2 healing methods of visualisation and colour healing. If you have a full length mirror, you can sit in front of it for this exercise. Don't worry if you haven't got one.

I will explain the mirror technique first, then go through the visualisation method.

Take some deep breaths, allow yourself to relax and your mind to settle.

Sit or stand in front of a mirror, look at yourself, you may visually see or imagine a colour surrounding you. If you are imagining a colour start by visualising a white colour surrounding you. White is a cleansing and protective colour, that can help with dissolving negativity.

You may feel the colour too, you may feel warmth or a coolness surrounding you. Keep that white healing light surrounding you for a few minutes.

Take some more deep breaths, and see in the mirror the colour of the white change to another healing colour. It could be gold which symbolizes, transformation, optimism and confidence. It could be blue which represents inner peace, security, tranquillity. Whichever colour you feel has a healing effect on you, see or feel it around you.

See the colour getting brighter and brighter, healing every level of your mind, body and soul.

Now to add some extra healing, see and feel if you can, some healing words in the colour surrounding you. You could see protection, strength, love, happiness, health etc. Take some deep breaths and try and feel these words around you, with each breath in the feeling of healing gets stronger, when you breath out your releasing anything you don't need.

Fill your aura full of healing words and feelings, and keep this image for a few minutes.

Practice this exercise when you feel like your aura is being affected by your own negative thoughts, feelings and emotions, or if you feel your being affected by your environment or other people's negativity.

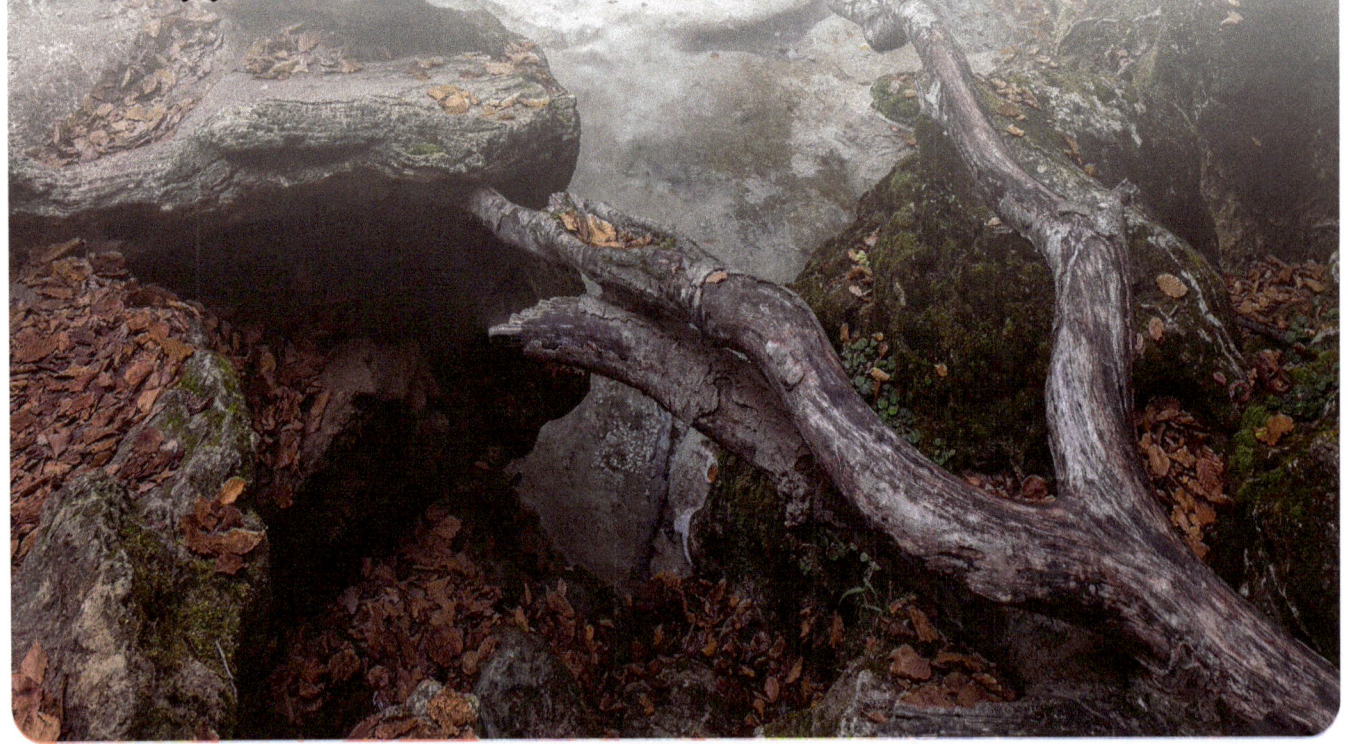

# Visualisation

Visualising is something that can help your mind through powerful imagery. Your mind can't tell if an image in your mind is real or not, so visualising what you want can help on so many subjects including; health, wealth, career, relationships etc.

Below is my visualisation script to help change negative feelings into positive ones. Please feel free to record it, so you can listen to it when you need.

> Take some deep breaths, and close your eyes. If any negative thoughts or emotions pop into your mind, imagine a dark stormy sky, all the negative thoughts, feelings, emotions and memories you feel is projected into the stormy sky.
>
> Observe what you're feeling and seeing, but don't dwell or go into a spiral of negativity.
>
> Take some deep breaths, and visualise the sun coming through the dark sky. With each of the sun's rays dissolving all negative words, thoughts, feeling and memories.
>
> See the dark sky turn blue with the sun still shining. See and feel positive words, memories, thoughts and feelings projected into the blue sky. Each time you breath in, the sky turns brighter and you feel calmer and more positive. With each breath out, you release all negativity you feel.
>
> Allow the healing to flow, with your mind full of peace and positivity. Keep this vision of the healing blue sky and positivity for as long as you can.
>
> Keep doing this visual exercise when you feel you need a lift in mood.

# Visualisation Method

Now I am going to go through the visualisation method. It's quite similar to the mirror method, but there will be no mirror and you're going to be closing your eyes.

Take some deep breaths, allow yourself to relax and let your mind settle.

Sit or lie down and close your eyes. In your mind visualize a healing colour, like white for cleansing and protection surrounding your whole body.

Start visualising the white colour, dissolving any negativity that you might be feeling or thinking, clearing away any unwanted energies around you.

Keep the white colour in your mind for a few minutes, then take some more deep breaths.

See in your mind the colour changing around you from white, to a healing colour. This could be gold, blue, green for balance growth and health.

Whichever colour your drawn to, let it surround your entire body from head to toe. See the colour getting brighter and brighter, healing you on every level of your mind, body and soul.

Now begin adding some healing words into your aura. Try and see and feel the words. You could add love, health, strength, peace, calm, happiness etc.

Take some deep breaths, and feel those words you have chosen. With each breath in, the feeling of healing gets stronger.

When you breath out, your releasing everything you don't need.

Fill your aura with healing words and feelings for a few minutes.

Keep practicing this method, when you feel like your aura or energy is being affected by negativity.

# Writing Your Own Visualisation Script

You can write your own visualisation script to help on any subject, including grief, negativity release, reaching goals and much more. Make sure that if you start feeling negative, to change the picture in your mind to create a shift in your thinking, to move your mind onto something positive.

Below is an example script that I have written to help with grief. Please feel free to record or use this visualisation when you need it.

> Take some deep breaths, close your eyes and see in your mind, that you are walking through a forest. Its chucking it down with rain, and you're carrying a heavy rucksack on your back filled with rocks. The rocks represent the grief, pain and sadness you're carrying around with you.
>
> As you walk through the forest, the rain slows and you see a stream of water. You take off the rucksack and sit on a log next to the stream. You take some deep breaths and allow your mind to slow and settle.
>
> You then walk over to the stream, and notice that the water is cleansing. It is water that releases pain and any feelings of hurt and sadness.
>
> You begin washing your hands and feet in the stream, allowing your mind, body and soul to bathe in the healing water, allowing all pain, sadness, grief and hurt your feeling to be washed away and released.

After spending some time in the healing stream, you open the rucksack and take out the rocks of grief, pain, sadness and hurt, placing them in the cleansing water. After a while the rocks begin to shrink into small pebbles.

Each pebble is infused full of love and healing energies, with a word written on each one. They are peace, comfort, strength and love. Hold these pebbles for a while to feel each healing word in your mind and heart.

You then put the pebbles in your bag and leave the forest with the sun shining, feeling able to be more at peace and being able to adjust and release all that you need.

You can create your own healing pebbles, by writing comforting words or quotes on them. You could place them around your home or somewhere that you see them often.

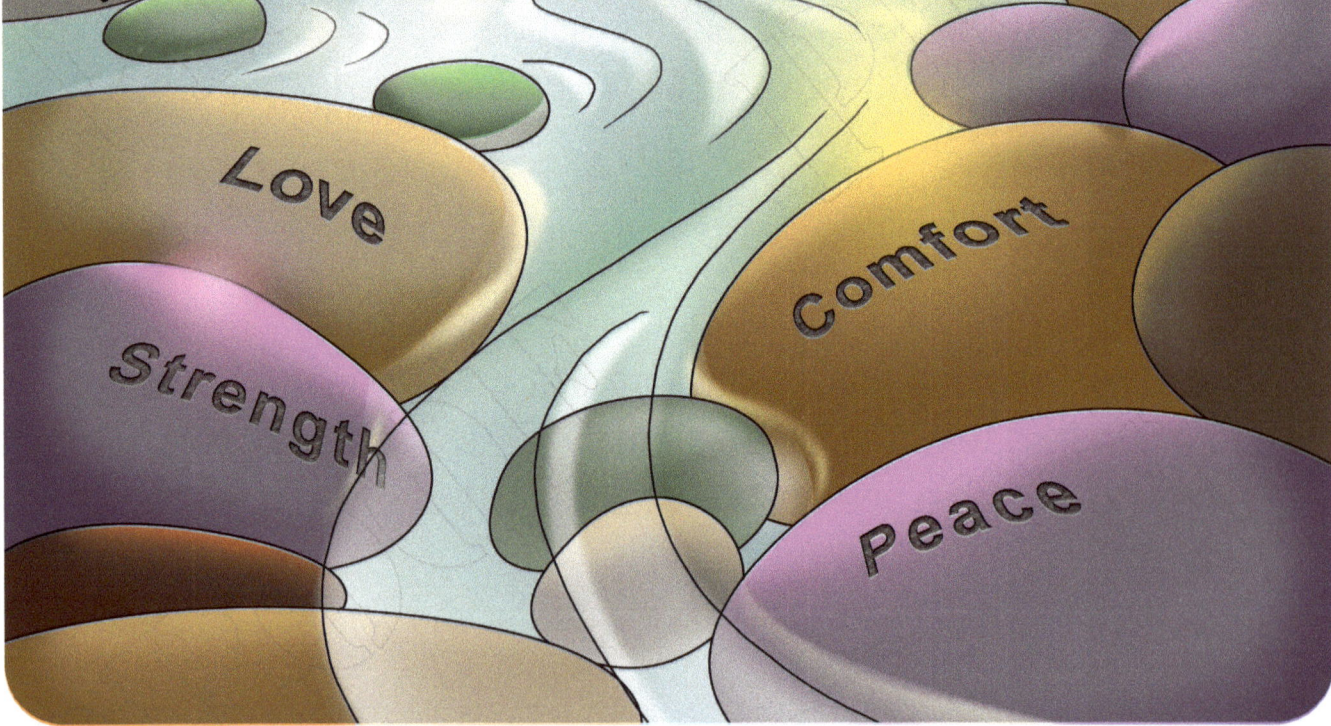

Mighty Mind Mantra's For Men

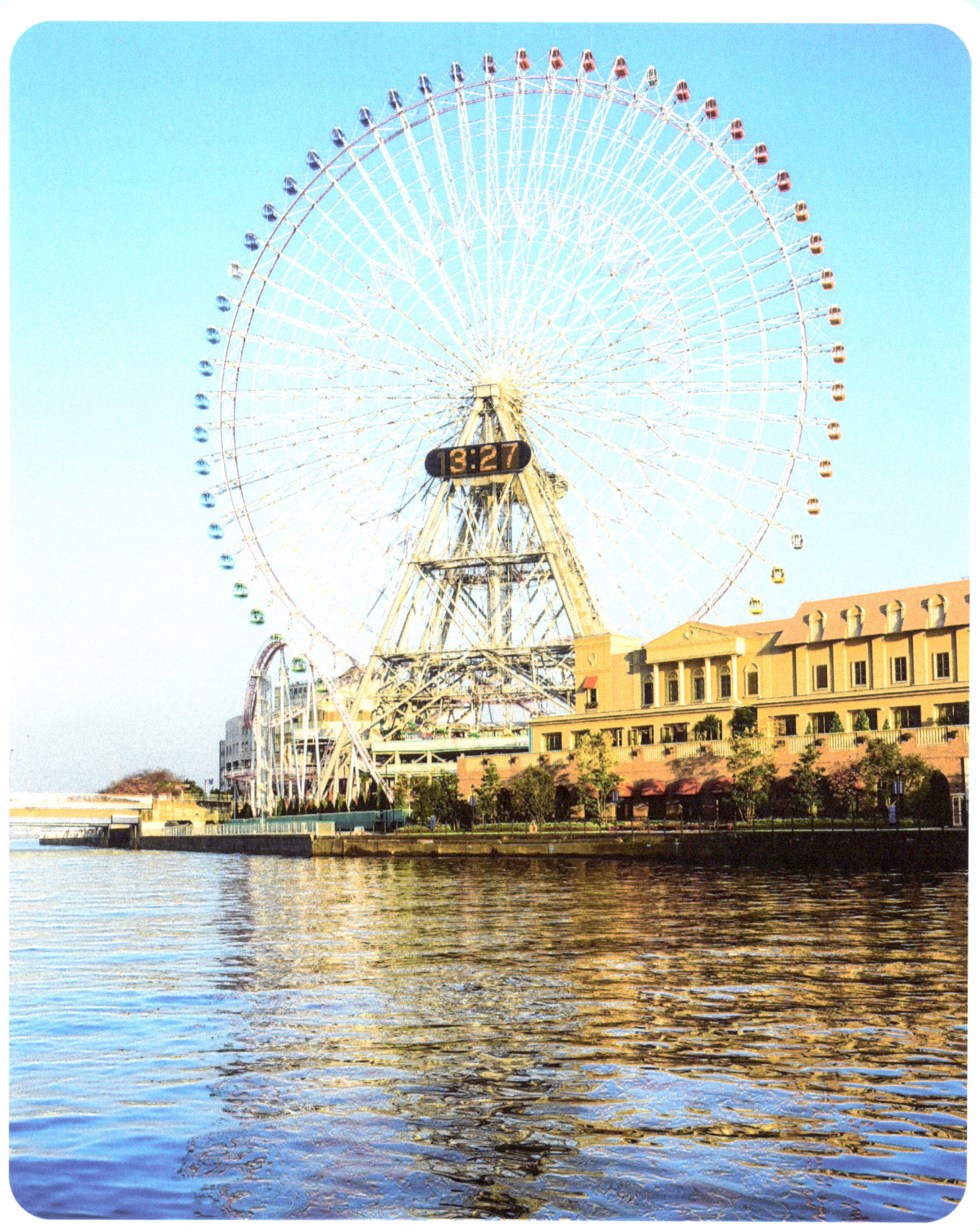

# Writing Your Own Visualisation Script

Now you can begin writing your own healing script on the next few pages. Remember to change a negative picture into a positive one. You can write a script about anything that you want to change.

_____
_____
_____
_____
_____
_____
_____
_____
_____
_____
_____
_____
_____
_____

Bella Hope Smith

# Mighty Mind Mantra's For Men

Bella Hope Smith

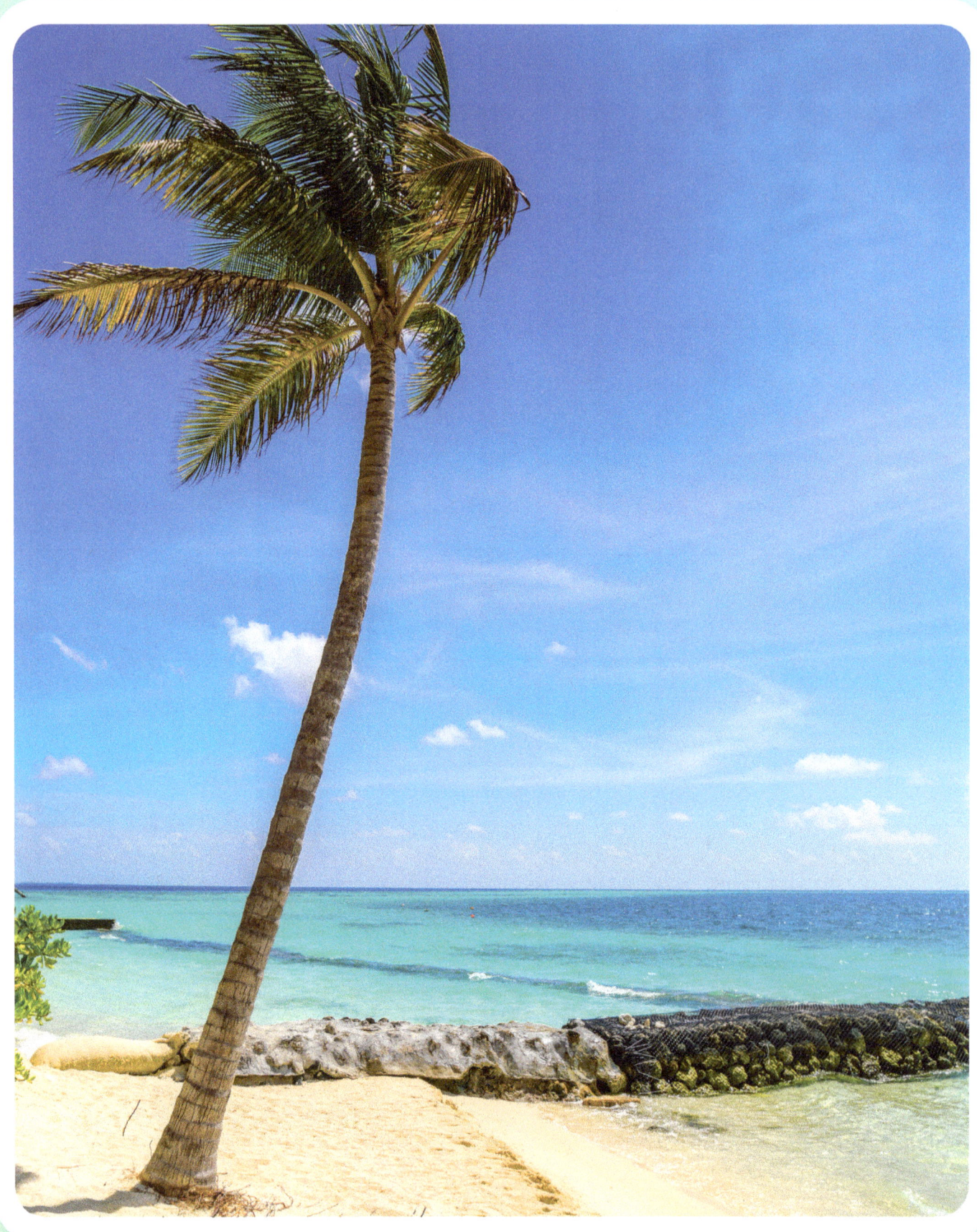

# Music Meditation

Music is very healing and therapeutic, and has lots of powerful benefits: including boosting the mood, relieving stress and relaxing the mind.

For the next exercise, I would like you to pick some music with lyrics. It could be rock, country, soul or any other genre you like.

Play the music and try and tune into the song, really listen to the lyrics, the rhythm and tempo. Take some deep breaths and check in with yourself with how the song is making you feel. You might feel sad, happy, joyful, relaxed. Music often triggers certain emotions, for example a song could be happy and upbeat, but you remember the song from an upsetting time in your life, so hearing it might trigger that memory causing you to feel sad.

After the song is finished, write down any words, memories, thoughts or feelings in the box below. This will help you connect with your emotions and feelings through music.

Now I want you to choose some music with no lyrics, just sound. Take some deep breaths, play the music and tune into the sound and rhythm of it. Notice how you're feeling whilst listening, and write in the box any words, memories, thoughts or feelings you get.

After you have done both exercises, compare both the way you felt listening to a song with lyrics, and how you felt just listening to pure music. Which did you feel helped you more? Did you release any emotions whilst listening the music? Write in the box below.

# Mighty Mind Mantra's

Now we are going to create some mighty mind mantra's, to help change your thought pattern into a more productive and positive one. There are lots of benefits to saying, thinking, writing or chanting mantra's, including: Helping to relieve stress, calming the mind and body and relaxing the immune system.

On the next few pages, I am going to share my mantra's I have written. You can use any of these to say, write, think or chant. Remember to repeat them as often as you can, this will start creating a healing seed in your mind, the more you use the mantra's, the more the seed will grow and blossom into a mighty mind. It takes on average 21 days to create a habit, so keep the mantra's going!

All of my mantra's are rhymed because rhyming has a certain pattern to it, where the brain can pick up the healing message quicker and easier. Rhyming also helps with neurodiverse minds too.

Below are a couple of rhyming reminders I have written, to help you feel better about how you feel.

- Never feel embarassed about how your feeling, there is absolutely no shame. Healing and happiness is everyone's biggest aim.

- Everyone makes mistakes, so don't worry and despair. Apologising and owning up, shows that you are truly sorry and care.

I now unlock deep emotions that have been hurting my heart. Writing and talking about how I feel, allows the healing to start.

I am ready to move forward in a practical and positive way. I am going to stay determind and motivated every single day.

I make a routine to read, write and rest. I take time out for myself, to build back to being my best

Healing and happiness starts from within. I am now ready for my wellbeing journey to begin.

I am proud of the person I am. I do everything the best that I can.

Expressing how I feel, allows me to be free and heal.

Judging is just another persons opinion or view. I cannot change what others say or do.

I am brave, I am strong, I am worthy, I belong.

Keeping my thoughts balanced and in control, helps me focus on my life. Making me determined to reach all my goals.

I deserve to be happy, healthy and totally at peace. Any thoughts that are holding me back, I now fully release.

I am a light in the dark. I am here to make my mark.

I am ready to heal, I have nothing to hide. I release all my feelings that I have kept bottled up inside.

My thoughts are calm, my body feels lighter. My mind is positive, I feel much brighter.

Forgiveness can be tough, but I want to move through the pain. I want a happy mind, not one of hate, bitterness and blame.

Bella Hope Smith

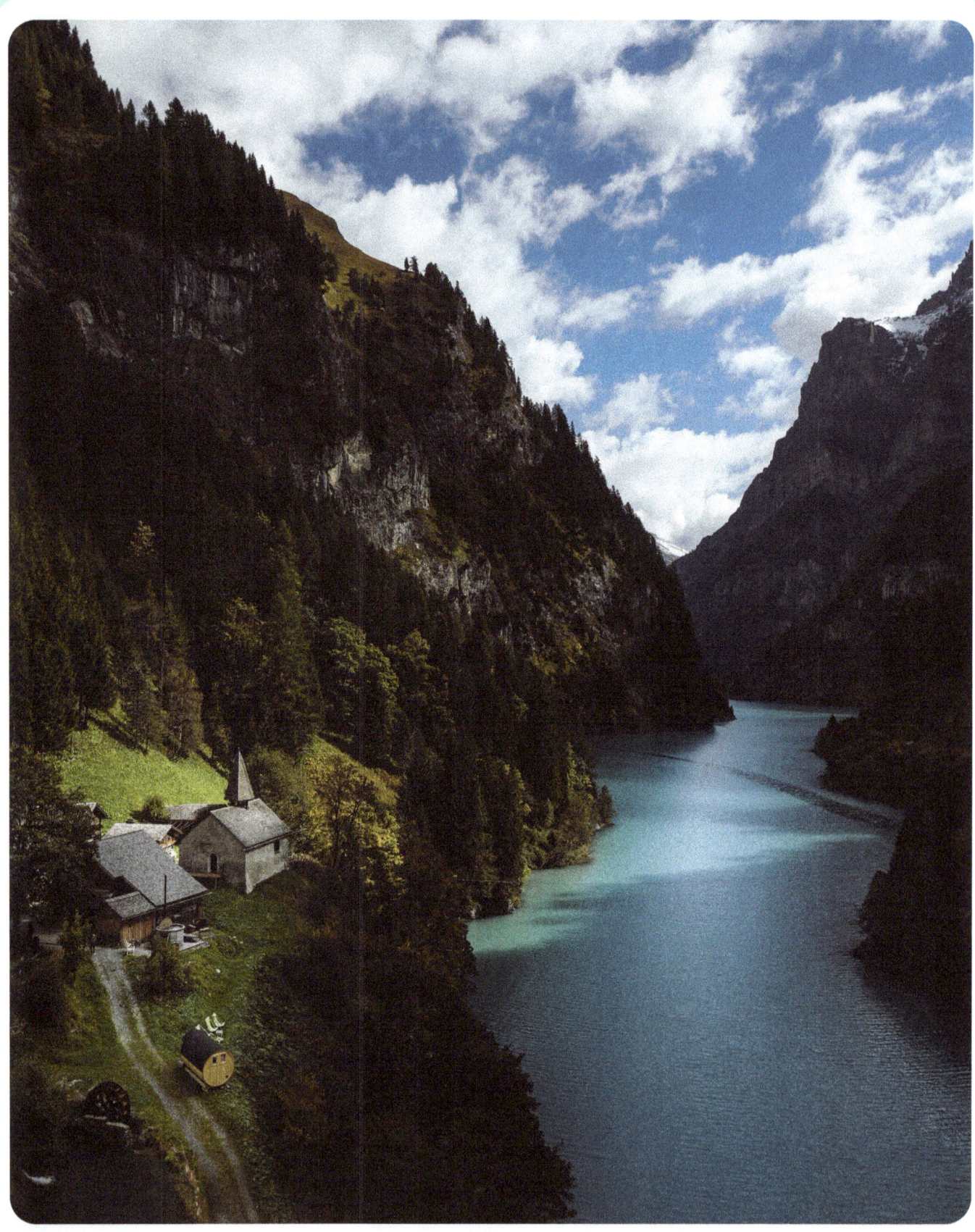

# Creating Your Own Mighty Mantra's

Firstly, it is best to choose an area that you need an extra boost of positivity or healing in. This could be health, wealth, relationships etc.

Next write a few words on how you would feel if you had that desired outcome. This could be happy, grateful, excited etc.

Here is my example below using the method. I am going to choose to write my mantra about **Health** and the words I would feel if I had better health would be, **Happy & Grateful**.

Now I will write a mantra using the topic of health and the 2 words of **Happy & Grateful**.

"I am happy and grateful, that my body and mind is healthy."

I have written some starter sentences that you could use to start your mantra's off. In brackets are the areas that you could use the starter sentence for.

"I am now attracting……" **(Wealth)**

"I am fully focused on ……." **(Health)**

"My mind stays positive……" **(Feelings)**

"I am totally ready for……." **(Relationships)**

Another way you can start writing your mantra's, are by using how you feel currently about various subject areas, and using the opposite emotion to create a positive mantra.

For example, if you feel disappointed because you're not making enough money, you look for the opposite word/ feeling to disappointed, which is the feeling of contentment and being satisfied.

Now we are going to write a healing mantra using the 2 words of **content and satisfied**, to create the opposite healing feeling to being disappointed, creating a shift in your emotional state.

**"I feel satisfied and content knowing, that money and abundance is constantly flowing."**

Try and write some opposite emotion mantra's to create a powerful shift in how you're feeling.

If you feel upset or distressed, the opposite emotions to these are peaceful and comfort, so use the words peaceful and comfort in your mantra.

If you feel doubtful or pessimistic, the opposite emotions to these are hopeful and faith, so use the words hopeful and faith in your mantra.

_____
_____
_____
_____
_____
_____
_____

# Creating Rhyming Mantra's

Firstly, I will write some start starter sentences that you can use to begin your mantra's.

- I feel positive about…….

- I keep my thoughts…….

- I express how I feel……

- I am ready for………

- My life is………

Next, we need some rhyming words to add into the mantra. I have written a list below that you can use.

- Healing, Feeling, Achieving, Dealing, Believing, Appealing, Receiving

- Right, Might, Night, Sight, Light, Bright, Delight, Alright

- Ground, Sound, Around, Found, Surround, Profound

- Proud, Crowd, Vowed, Cloud, Allowed

- Success, Bless, Access, Dress

- New, View, Do, Too

- Me, Be, Tree, See, Free

If you have your own list of rhyming words, you can write them in the box below.

Now we are going to put everything together to create a mighty mantra. I am going to choose the starter sentence; **"I am ready for"** and I am going to choose the 2 rhyming words of **Success and Dress**.

Below is my example mantra.

"I am ready for my life to change into one of happiness and success. I am proud of myself, from my kind personality to the way I look and dress".

If you are finding it a bit tricky to create some rhyming mantra's, then here are some mantra sentences with the last 2 words left blank for you to add in the rhyming words. You can use words from the rhyming list, or your own rhyming words.

I am now ready to start……………………….. I feel proud of myself and what I am …………………………

Healing is happening, I see it all ………………….. Love and peace is what I have ……………………………

Abundance flows easily and effortlessly to …………… Which makes me happy and ……………………..

Everything will get better, it will be …………………….. Healing is surrounding me every day and every …………..

I am trying to process how I am ……………………… I allow my thoughts to be ones of hope, happiness and …………………

On the next few pages, you can write down your mighty mantra's

Mighty Mind Mantra's For Men

Bella Hope Smith

Bella Hope Smith

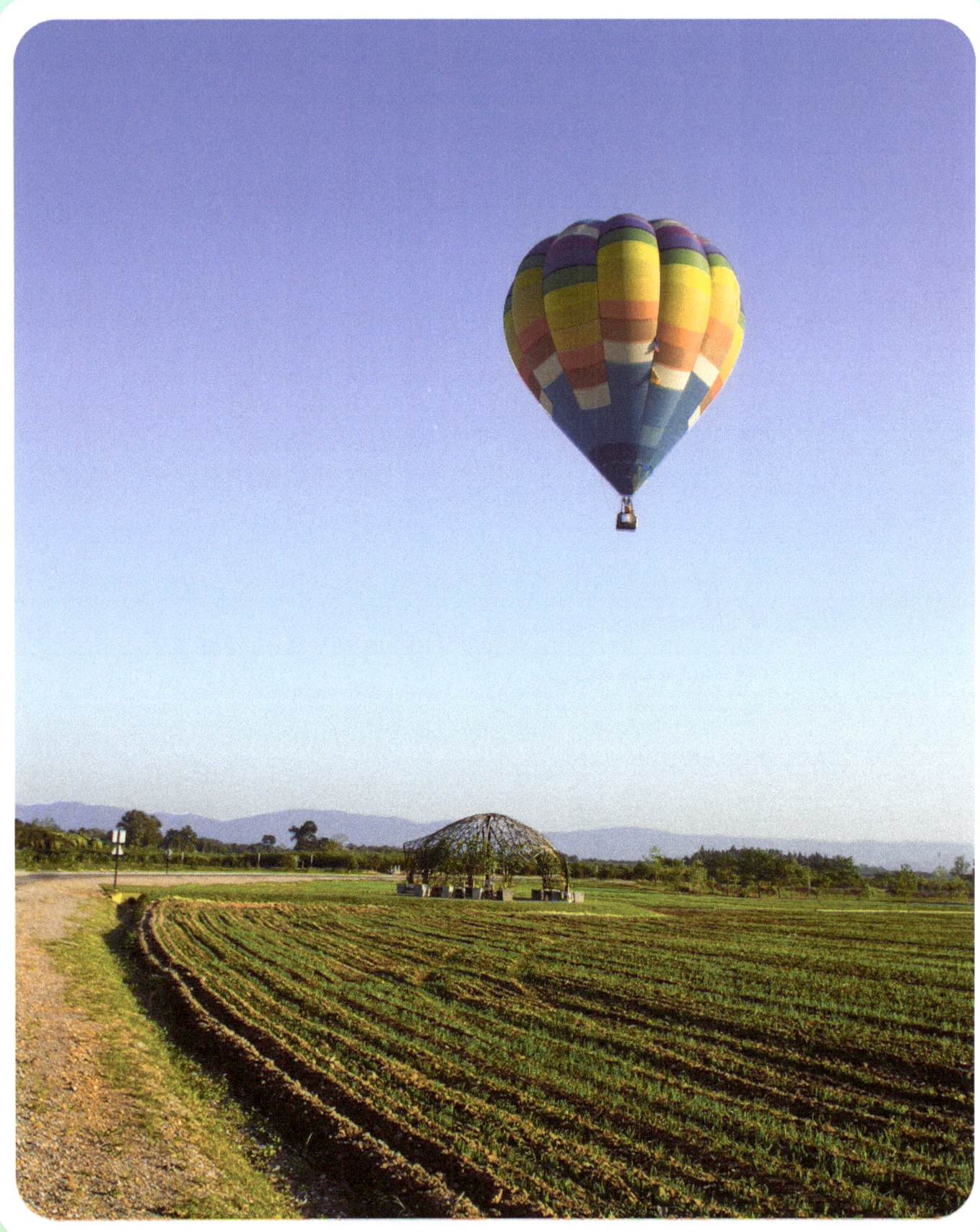

## The Benefits Of The Thymus Gland With Helping You Feel Calmer

The thymus gland is used to protect the immune system, and balance the hormones in the body. When the thymus gland is gently tapped, it can help calm anxiety and relax the body. When you first tap this gland, it may feel tender, but gently tapping the thymus overtime, will make the tenderness fade.

I am going to show you a technique you can use if you have said, written, read or thought anything sad or negative, which includes emotions such as blame, hate, bitterness, grief, anger etc.

**Below is a diagram on where you will find the thymus gland on your body.**

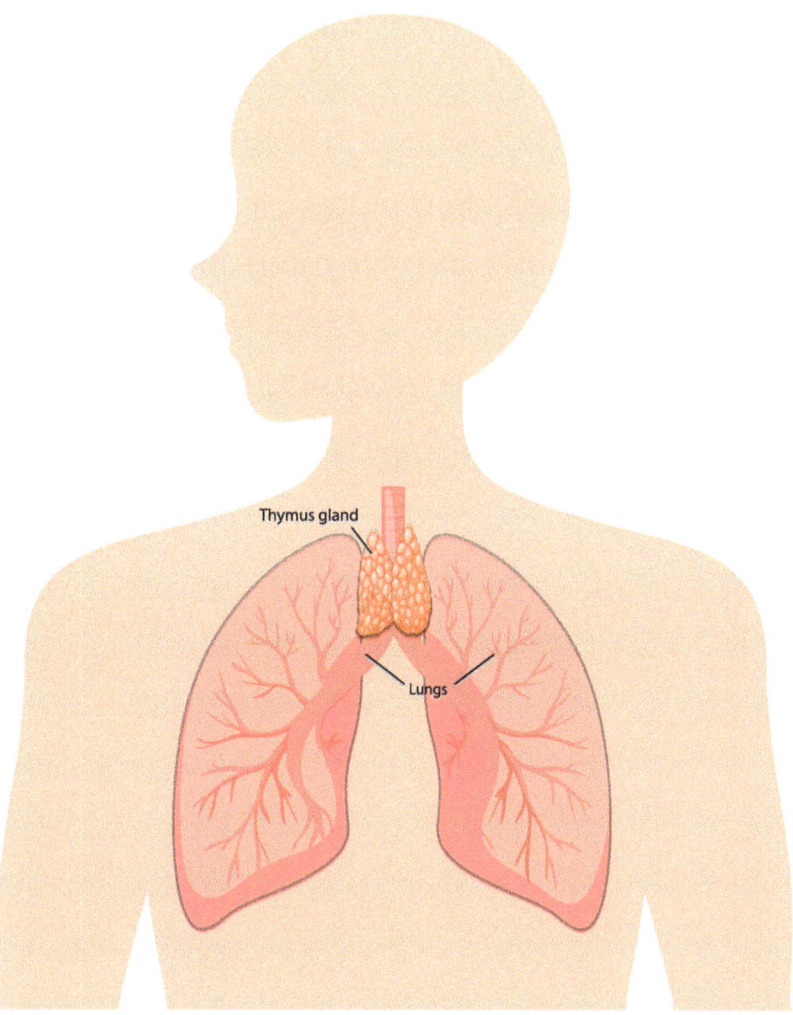

Now I am going to show you a technique you can use, when you feel anxious, stressed or negative.

Step 1. **Take some deep breaths, allow your body to relax and your mind to slow.**

Step 2. **If you have written, thought or said anything negative or upsetting, I want you to clap your hands or listen to drumming music, whilst taking more deep breaths.**

The reason I say clap or listen to drumming music, is sound therapy breaks up stuck and unwanted energies, allowing room for healing vibrations to flow in. After you have finished clapping or listening to drums, you might feel a sense of relaxation or calm.

Step 3. **Start gently tapping the thymus gland for around 15-30 seconds. Whilst tapping visualise a healing image in your mind. It could be a place that you love, and keep that image in your mind whilst tapping and for a few minutes after you have stopped tapping. Let the image gradually fade and take some more deep breaths.**

Step 4. **Now place your hand on your heart, and say out loud or in your mind a positive word or one of the mighty mantra's, either your own mantra or one of mine from the list. Keep reciting the mantra until you feel a shift in your feelings and thoughts.**

Keep doing this technique everytime you need to feel calmer and more relaxed. Tapping your thymus will give your immune system a boost too.

## Gratitude In Steps

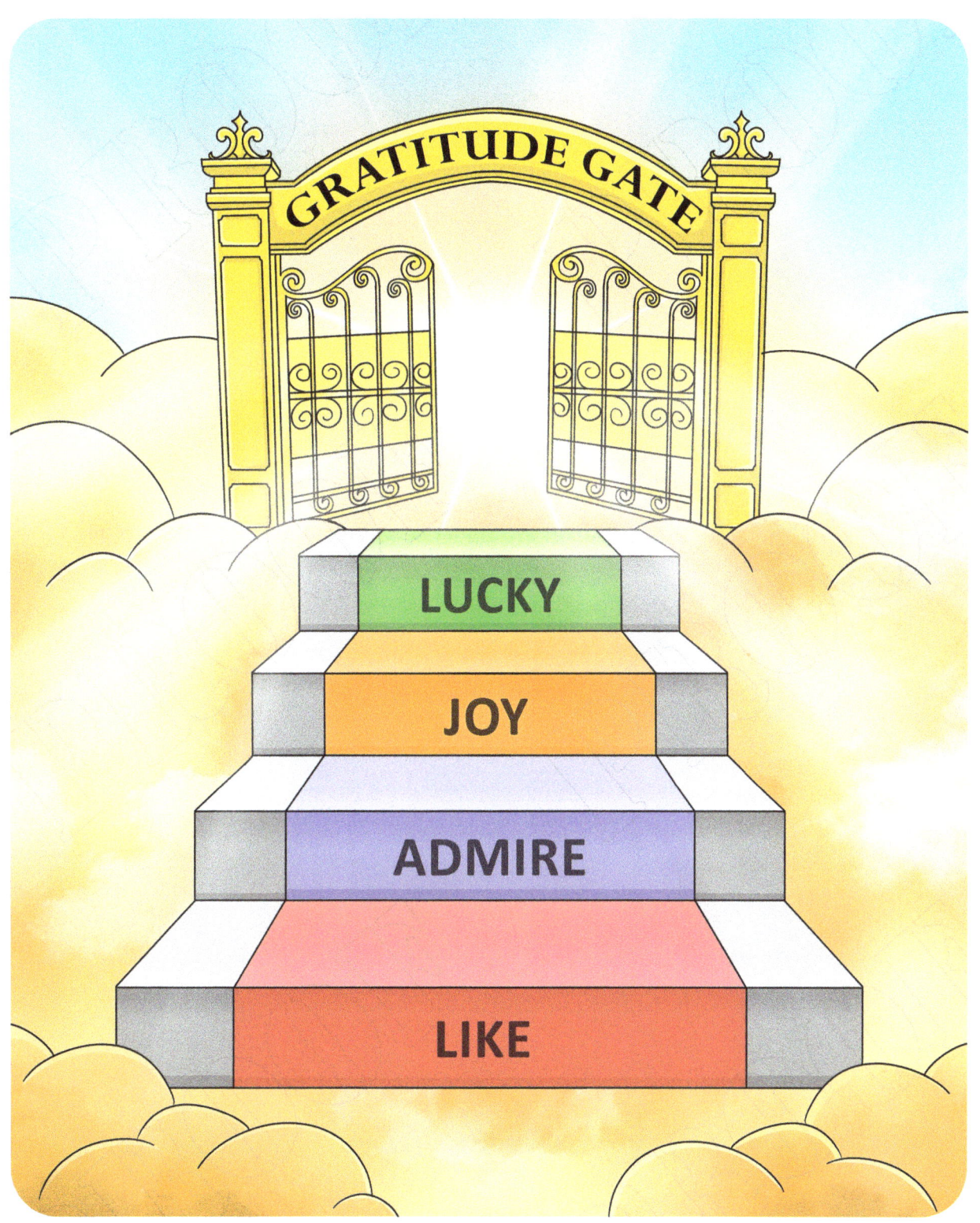

Gratitude is such a big word, that often we sometimes struggle to find things to be grateful for when times are tough.

I am going to show you my technique to help you build up to an attitude of gratitude in small steps.

Remember there is no rush on moving through all the steps at once, only move onto the next step when you feel ready to do so.

The first word on the steps we are going to use, is the word **Like**. I want you to begin writing down over the next few days, things that you like. Some examples could be "I like this song" or "I like this food" etc. You will be surprised on how many things you like.

_____

_____

_____

_____

_____

_____

_____

_____

_____

Mighty Mind Mantra's For Men

Bella Hope Smith

# Mighty Mind Mantra's For Men

Now write in the box below how you felt after doing this exercise. Did you find it easy/difficult?

After you're ready move onto the next step, we are going to write about things that you **Admire**. Again, start writing even if it is for 2 or 3 days, things you admire. Some examples could be "I admire a personality trait in myself" or someone else or "I admire this beautiful scenery" etc.

_____
_____
_____
_____
_____
_____
_____
_____
_____
_____
_____
_____
_____
_____
_____
_____
_____
_____

Bella Hope Smith

Mighty Mind Mantra's For Men

Now write in the box below how you felt after doing this exercise. Did you find it easy/difficult? Did it help you focus your mind on something more positive? How did it make you feel?

After you're ready to move onto the 3rd step, we are going to write about things that bring you **Joy**. Some examples could be "I feel joy listening to music" or "I feel joy watching sport" etc.

_____
_____
_____
_____
_____
_____
_____
_____
_____
_____
_____
_____
_____
_____
_____
_____

Again, begin writing in the box how you feel writing about things that bring you joy. Did you find it easy/difficult? Did it help you focus your mind on something more positive? How did it make you feel?

When you're ready to move onto the next step, we are going to write about things you feel **Lucky** for. Some examples could be "I feel lucky to have caring people in my life" or "I feel lucky that I can read and write" etc.

Mighty Mind Mantra's For Men

Now write in the box below how you felt after doing this exercise.

When you are totally ready to move on, we are going to arrive at the gates of **Gratitude**.

Remember it can take a while to feel gratitude, so don't be hard on yourself if you don't feel that straight away. If you don't feel ready to write about gratitude, don't worry just go back to any of the gratitude steps, and try and build from there.

Here are some examples you could write about. "I am grateful that I can see/hear/walk/talk" or "I am grateful for my health" etc

_____
_____
_____
_____
_____
_____
_____
_____
_____
_____
_____
_____
_____
_____

# Mighty Mind Mantra's For Men

Bella Hope Smith

Mighty Mind Mantra's For Men

Bella Hope Smith

After you have written about gratitude, write in the box how it made you feel, plus how doing the whole exercise made you feel. Do you feel a shift in your mindset? Do you feel a sense of calm or peace after writing about positive things?

Try and do this exercise regularly, to help keep an optimistic view and a mighty mindset.

# Creating Your Own Gratitude Steps

Below are some steps left blank that I want you to write your own healing words in, to get to the great gates of gratitude. I have put some example words below to help you.

- Favourite
- Blessed
- Passionate
- Love

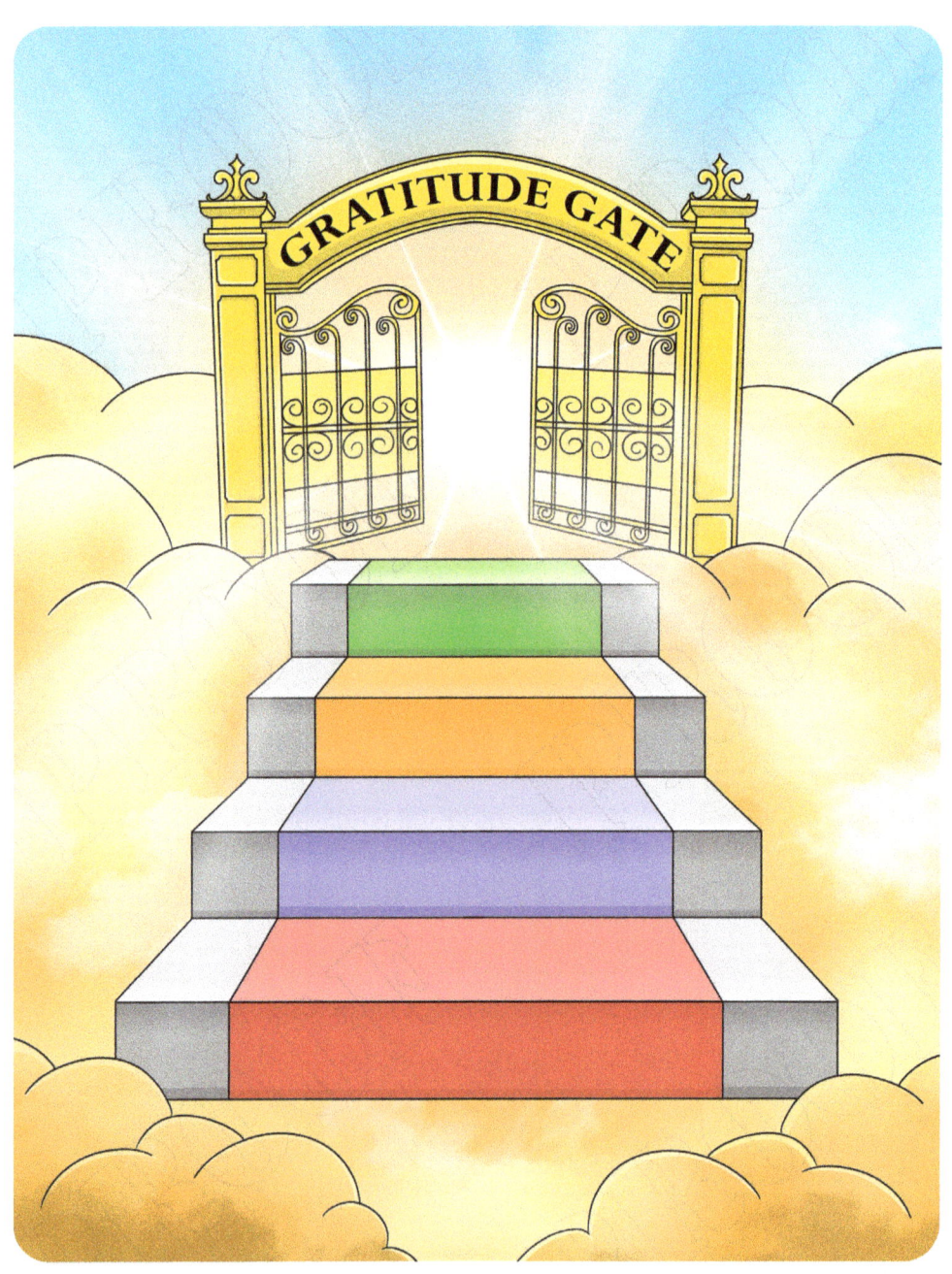

Now begin following the same method as before, and write in the boxes after each step how you feel.

Mighty Mind Mantra's For Men

Now write in the box below how you felt after doing the exercise. Did you find it easy/difficult?

# Mighty Mind Mantra's For Men

How did you feel after doing this exercise? Did you find it easy/difficult?

Mighty Mind Mantra's For Men

Bella Hope Smith

# Mighty Mind Mantra's For Men

How did you feel after doing this exercise? Did you find it easy/difficult?

Mighty Mind Mantra's For Men

How did you feel after doing this exercise? Did you find it easy/difficult?

Mighty Mind Mantra's For Men

Bella Hope Smith

Mighty Mind Mantra's For Men

How did you feel doing this exercise? Did you find it easy/difficult?

# Learning Something New

We are now going to look into different areas to help your mind focus on something that you're interested in doing or learning, by creating a more optimistic point of view using the gratitude steps, and the mighty mantra's. It will help you to focus on all the good and new things that life has to offer.

First, I would like you to write down areas, subjects, things that interest you, or something that you want to learn. I have given some examples that you could write below.

- I want to learn a new language.
- I want to learn to play an instrument.
- I want to learn to sing/rap.
- I am interested in photography.
- I am interested in drawing.
- I would love to become a life coach.

When you have written a list, we are going to turn them into a mighty mantra to help your mind focus on your desired outcome. It will keep you motivated and determined to reach your goal.

First, we are going to choose an emotion, on how you would feel if you achieved or begin learning something new. Examples – **Excitement, Happiness, Proud.**

Next, we are going to use the emotions you would feel in your mighty mantra.

Here is my example below using the words, **Excitement, Happiness & Proud.**

"I feel proud of myself for learning something new. Happiness and excitement fill my mind with what I can now do"

Write as many mantra's as you like to help keep your mind focused on something you want to do and achieve.

# Mighty Mind Mantra's For Men

After you feel more confident in reaching your desired outcome, we are going to turn it into action.

Write down some ways on how you could achieve your goal.

I have written down some examples on what you could do
- Buy a book on what you want to learn about
- Watch videos or tutorials online on how to do something
- Look out for any classes or groups you could join in person or online
- Connect with like-minded people on forums or online communities, that also share your interests and passions
- Go to a library to read or use their facilities to learn about your chosen subjects

_____
_____
_____
_____
_____
_____
_____
_____
_____

Following all the steps, will help keep your mind on something you want to achieve. It helps your mental health, as your keeping focused on your goal with mantra's and your acting on getting what you want.

Bella Hope Smith

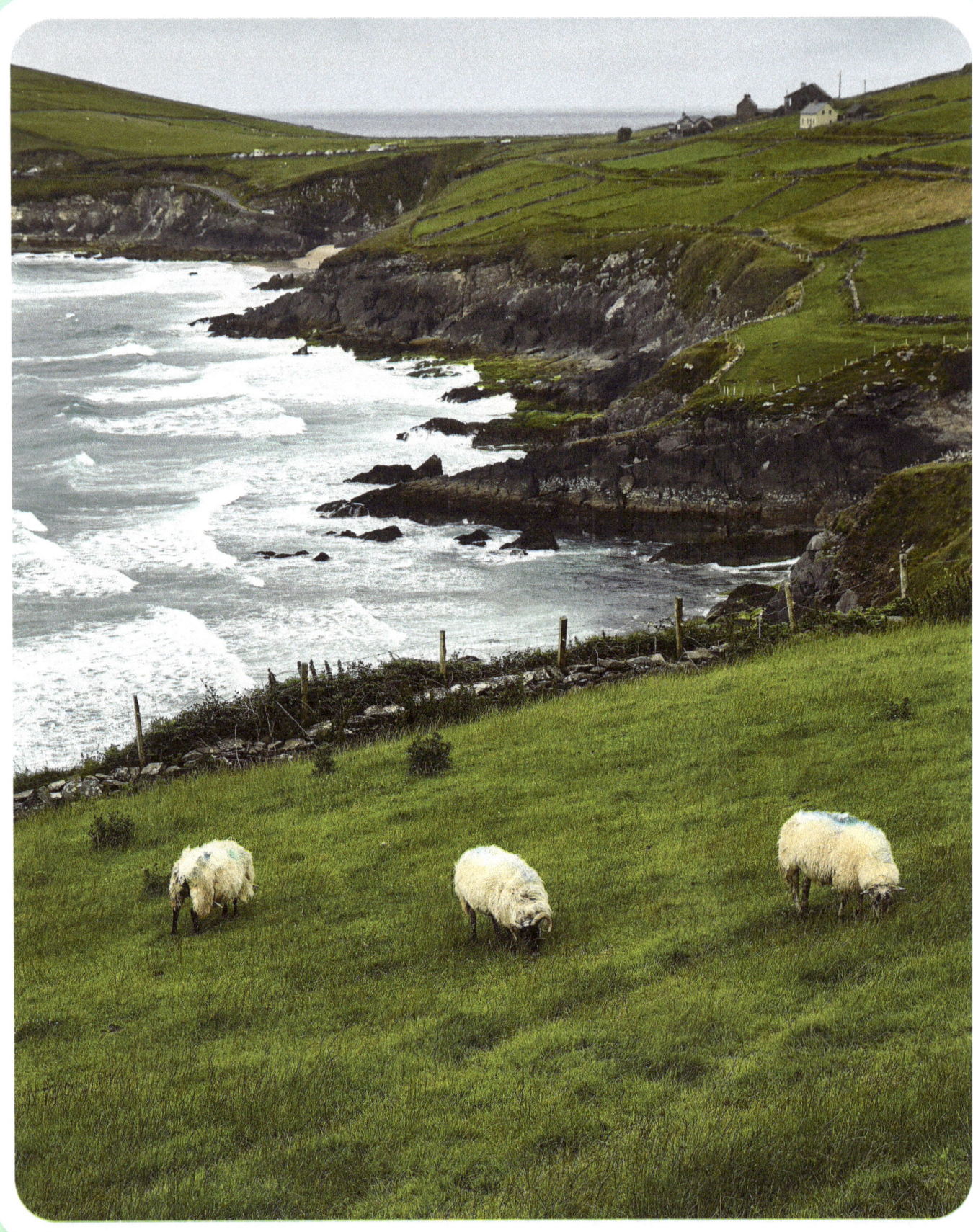

# Volunteering

I wanted to mention about all the benefits there are to volunteering. Here are just a few below.

- Builds confidence
- Helping a worthy cause
- Making new friends
- Having faith and belief in yourself
- Learning new things
- Focuses your mind on something positive
- Making a change

If you were interested in volunteering in person or virtually, there are a lot of different foundations, charities and groups you can choose from. If you are looking to help out or volunteer, choose an area that is close to your heart or are passionate about helping. It could be helping animals, helping people mentally/physically/emotionally, it could be helping at a museum, art centre or in your local community. Research about areas your interested in with volunteering, create a mighty mantra to focus on the goal of volunteering, write what emotions you would feel if you're helping out, recite the mantra often, then act on your desired goal, just like the method on the previous page.

# Mighty Mind Mantra's For Men

Bella Hope Smith

# Word Puzzle To Help Your Mind

Puzzles can help reduce stress, problem solve, focus and engage the mind, which helps mental wellbeing.

## Scramble Word Game

Below are some words, where I want you to write as many new words out of them as you can.

For example, in the word **Seasoning**, I can make the words: Ago, Eon, Sea, Song, Gone etc.

Write down as many words that you can make out of

Affirmations

_____
_____
_____
_____
_____
_____

Resilience

_____
_____
_____

Breakthrough

Supportive

## Compassion

_____
_____
_____
_____
_____

## Therapeutic

_____
_____
_____
_____
_____

## Mindfulness

_____
_____
_____
_____
_____

Inspirational

Meditation

Forgiveness

## Excitement

## Achievement

# Holistic Healing

Below I have written a list of various natural and holistic therapies that work well alongside writing therapy. If you are interested in any of the therapies, thoroughly research it and remember to always seek help and advice from health professionals.

- Art Therapy
- Yoga
- Sound Therapy
- Animal Assisted Therapy
- Reiki
- Naturopathy
- Cognitive Behavioural Therapy
- Breathwork
- Laughter Yoga
- Tai Chi
- Herbal Medicine
- Aromatherapy
- Walking Meditation
- Reflexology
- Ayurveda

Mighty Mind Mantra's For Men

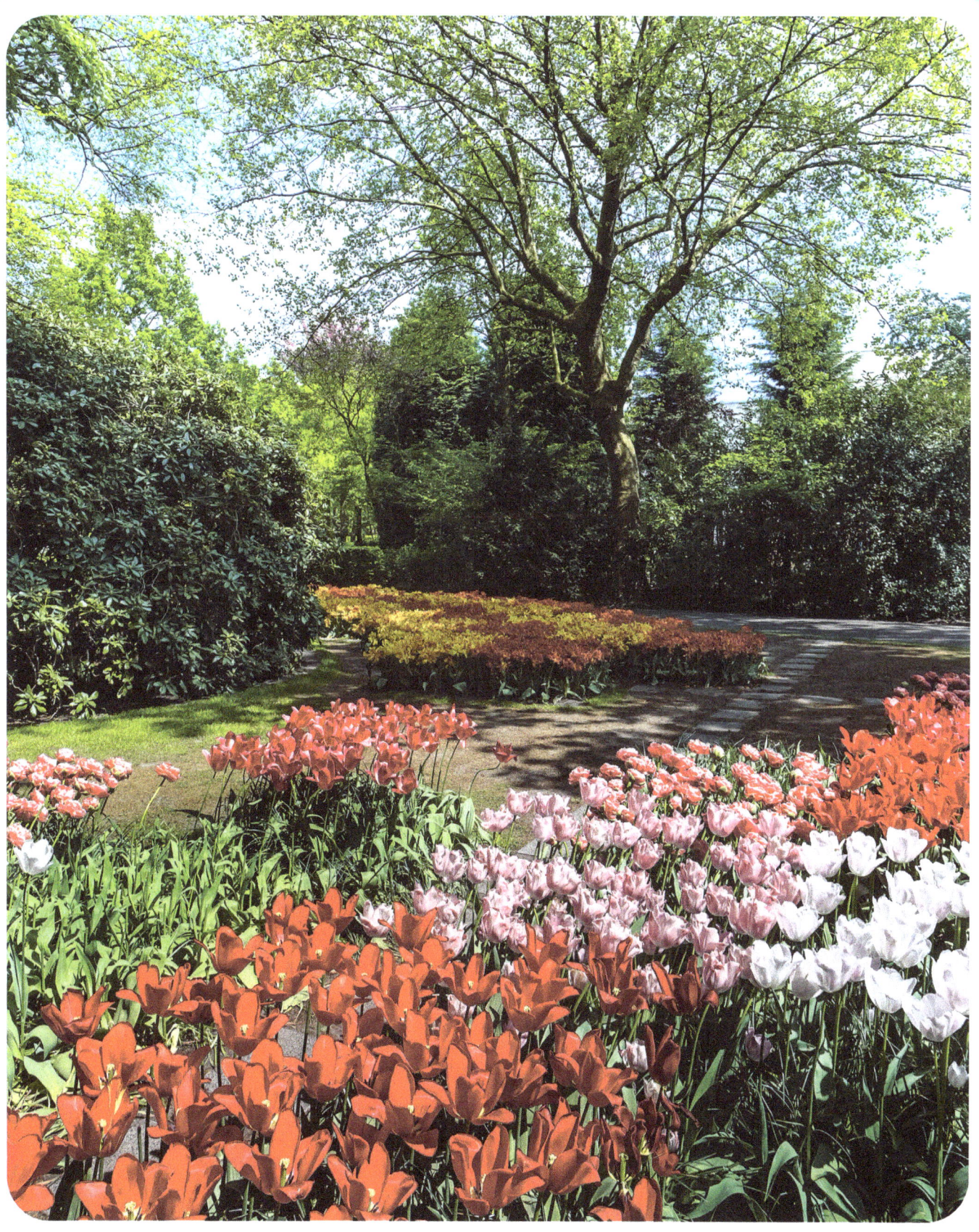

I hope my book has allowed you to express your feelings in different ways, and that you begin to start opening up to people when you need help, instead of keeping things to yourself causing you stress and worry. I hope your mental health starts to improve, with feelings of hope, healing and happiness filling your mind.

I thought I would finish on a few mighty mind mantra's that I would like you to always remember.

"Always remember there are people to help you, from a stranger to a friend. Things will get better and brighter in the end."

"Please don't hesitate or think twice, about asking for any help or advice."

"You are more loved and appreciated than you realise. You are wanted, worthy and wise."

"Practice a regular routine to let out your creativity. It will help you focus on something positive, instead of negativity."